Quiet the Food Noise

Transforming Your Relationship with Food Through Faith

NJ Domrufus

Gifted Anchor Books

Copyright © 2024 by Njideka Domrufus

All rights reserved.

No portion of this book may be reproduced in any form without written permission from the publisher or author, except as permitted by U.S. copyright law.

Gifted Anchor Books

ISBN: 9781965945230

Printed in the United States of America.

Dedication

To my mum, Your love, wisdom, and unwavering belief in me have been my guiding light. Thank you for always being my greatest support and inspiration. This book is for you.

Acknowledgements

Writing this book has been an incredible journey, and I am deeply grateful to everyone who has supported and believed in this message of faith and freedom.

First, I thank God for His guidance, strength, and grace throughout this process. Without Him, this book would not have been possible.

To my loving husband and two beautiful daughters—your unwavering support, prayers, and love mean everything to me. Thank you for giving me the space and encouragement to bring this vision to life.

To my pastor, our man of God Prophet Richard A. Gyamfi, thank you so much for always standing by us and for your prayers; and Bishop Samuel Boakye for all your help with editing, and making sure this book was published.

To my dear friends, readers, and clients—your stories and support have been a true blessing and inspiration. Thank you for trusting me with your journey.

Lastly, to you, the reader—thank you for your willingness to explore these ideas and embark on this journey. I hope these pages bring you comfort, strength, and a renewed connection with God.

With gratitude,

Dr. NJ Domrufus, DNP

Forward

Quiet the Food Noise: *Transforming Your Relationship with Food Through Faith* is a divine invitation to reclaim the joy and peace God intended for us through His gift of food. In a culture bombarded with diet trends, restrictive eating plans, and mixed messages about our bodies, Dr. NJ Domrufus offers something radically different. A Christ-centered approach to our relationship with food, rooted in the power of faith and freedom found in God's truth.

Dr. NJ Domrufus, with both professional insight and personal empathy, delves deep into the heart of what she terms "food noise." Grounded in faith, her approach draws upon biblical principles and spiritual wisdom to help readers break free from the unhealthy cycles that often accompany our eating habits. She does not merely guide readers toward better physical health; she presents a path to spiritual healing, emphasizing that our journey with food is intertwined with our journey of faith.

This book is not just about eating differently, it's about living differently; reclaiming our identity in Christ and stepping into the fullness of life He offers. With compassion, wisdom, and personal testimony, Dr. Domrufus reminds us that every meal is an opportunity to draw closer to God, to practice gratitude, and to celebrate the beautiful truth that we are "fearfully and wonderfully made."

As you turn these pages, may you find solace, guidance, and a renewed sense of purpose in your journey with food. Above all, may you embrace the profound truth that food, like all gifts from God, is meant to bring you closer to His peace, joy, and love. – Samuel Boakye.

Authors Note

In a world where messages about food and body image can be overwhelming and often conflicting, it's easy to feel trapped in a cycle of worry, guilt, and confusion. As a Christian and mental health professional, my deepest desire is to guide you toward a faith-centered, healthy relationship with food—one that brings peace instead of anxiety, freedom instead of guilt, and true fulfillment instead of emptiness.

This book is for anyone who has struggled with the constant "food noise"—the thoughts about what you should or shouldn't eat, whether you look "good enough," or if you're doing "enough" to be healthy. If you've felt burdened by these thoughts, please know you're not alone. I've walked this road myself, and I know that God never intended for us to be weighed down by these worries. Instead, He invites us to live in freedom, trusting that He has provided everything we need for both body and soul.

The journey to this freedom starts with the realization that food is not our enemy. It's a gift from God, meant to nourish us and bring joy—not to be a source of guilt or a way to cope with deeper struggles. Together, we'll explore the roots of our relationship with food, why we may overeat, and how to realign our motives in ways that honor both our bodies and our Creator.

In writing Quiet the Food Noise: *Transforming Your Relationship with Food Through Faith,* I've drawn from years of experience as a mental health provider, my personal faith journey, and my work with individuals who have wrestled with food noise. My hope is that through these pages, you'll find a path to freedom from unhealthy eating patterns and body image struggles. True hope and healing are within reach when we lean into God's truth, find strength in Him, and surround ourselves with support that lifts us up.

As you read, I hope you feel seen, understood, and encouraged. I hope you find practical tools, spiritual insights, and a sense of community that will support you in quieting the noise and discovering a renewed peace with food. Most importantly, I pray that you'll experience the freedom that comes from surrendering to God and letting Him transform your relationship with food.

Let's take this journey together—one of healing, hope, and finding peace in the noise. May you uncover faith, freedom, and a fresh sense of purpose as you turn each page.

Dr. NJ Domrufus, DNP

Contents

1. Introduction — 1
2. Biblical Perspective on Food and Eating — 4
3. Rethinking Eating Habits — 12
4. Breaking Free from Food Noise — 23
5. Fasting, Feasting, and Spiritual Health — 30
6. Fellowship, Accountability, and Mental Health — 41
7. Conclusion — 46
8. Appendices A - Quieting Food Noise: Daily Thought Record — 49
9. Appendices B - Daily Thought Record Worksheet — 63
10. Appendices C- Emotional Check-In Chart — 65
11. Appendices D- The 5-Minute Delay Technique — 67
12. Reference — 69

1

Introduction

Understanding Food Noise: Transforming Your Relationship with Food Through Faith

Welcome, friend. I'm grateful you're here and that you've chosen to embark on this journey. If you've ever felt consumed by thoughts about food—what to eat, when to eat, how much to eat—know that you're not alone. I call this constant mental chatter "food noise." It's that background buzz that can distract you from living fully and serving God wholeheartedly. Food noise often pulls us away from our peace, our faith, and the freedom God desires for us. But here's the encouraging news: it doesn't have to be this way. With God's help, we can quiet this noise and discover true freedom.

As a Christian and a mental health professional, I've witnessed how struggles with food impact every part of a person's life—not only their physical health but also their emotional and spiritual well-being. Many people feel trapped, anxious, or even ashamed, believing they're alone in this battle. But nothing could be further from the truth. God cares deeply about every part of your life, including your relationship with food.

This book is an invitation to understand food noise—what it is, where it stems from, and how we can rise above it with faith. Together, we'll delve into biblical truths, practical tools, and spiritual disciplines that can guide you toward a peaceful, grace-filled relationship with food. This journey isn't about quick fixes or the latest diet trends. It's about embracing a new way of thinking, one that leads to lasting transformation—a way that honors God and brings the freedom and peace you've been longing for.

At the end of the book, you'll find practical tools to support this journey, including Activities and Worksheets designed to help you quiet food noise and manage cravings. These include:

- *Quieting Food Noise: Daily Thought Record*
- *Managing Cravings: The 5-Minute Delay Technique*
- *Overcoming Emotional Eating: Emotional Check-In Chart*

These tools will help you put what you've learned into practice, empowering you to take intentional steps toward peace and freedom. Let's walk this journey together, with open hearts and a readiness to find renewed purpose and joy.

What is Food Noise?

Food noise is that constant mental preoccupation with eating. It can manifest as worries about calories, obsessive thoughts about what you'll eat next, or guilt about what you've eaten in the past. Food noise can come from many sources—diet culture, past trauma, stress, or even well-meaning advice from others. It creates a cycle that keeps us bound and distracted, taking up precious mental space that could be used to grow closer to God, nurture relationships, and fulfill our purpose.

> God did not design us to live in bondage—not to sin, not to fear, and certainly not to food. In John 10:10, Jesus says, *"I have come that they may have life, and have it to the full."*

Food noise robs us of this fullness. It takes something that God created as good—nourishment and enjoyment—and twists it into a source of anxiety and shame. But God has a different plan for us, one that involves freedom, joy, and peace.

Finding Faith and Freedom

The journey to quieting food noise begins with faith. Faith that God cares about your struggles, faith that you are not alone, and faith that with His help, change is possible. In Romans 12:2, we are told, "*Do not conform to the pattern of this world, but be transformed by the renewing of your mind.*" This transformation isn't just about what we eat or how much we eat—it's about renewing our minds to think differently about food, our bodies, and our worth.

Throughout this book, we'll explore how to replace the lies that food noise tells us with God's truth. We'll talk about practical ways to approach eating with grace, how to identify the emotional and spiritual roots of food struggles, and how to bring those struggles before God. We'll also learn how to use spiritual disciplines like prayer, fasting, and fellowship to find true freedom.

This journey won't always be easy, but it will be worth it. As you begin this process, I want you to know that God sees you, He loves you, and He is ready to walk alongside you. You are not in this alone. Together, we will learn to quiet the food noise, find peace, and live in the freedom that Christ has promised us.

So, take a deep breath, grab a cup of tea, and let's begin this journey together. It's time to quiet the noise and embrace the abundant life God has for you.

2—

Biblical Perspective on Food and Eating

God's Design and Wisdom

Food is a gift from God, created with a specific purpose in mind. In Genesis 1:29-30, God says, *"I give you every seed-bearing plant on the face of the whole earth and every tree that has fruit with seed in it. They will be yours for food."* This verse reminds us that food was part of God's original plan—a means to sustain life, nourish our bodies, and fulfill His purpose for creation. To truly understand the purpose of food, we need to look at the intent of our Creator, just as we would look at the manufacturer's instructions to understand the purpose of a product.

God designed food not just to fill our stomachs, but to be an integral part of our well-being. He embedded within creation the nutrients and sustenance we need for our bodies to thrive. Food is part of a divine system, where every plant, animal, and nutrient play a role in supporting life. When we view food in this way—as a gift from our loving Creator—we begin to understand its significance beyond mere sustenance.

Nourishment in Scripture

Food serves a purpose far beyond satisfying hunger; it is an essential part of God's design for our well-being. Psalm 104:14-15 says, "*He makes grass grow for the cattle, and plants for people to cultivate—bringing forth food from the earth: wine that gladdens human hearts, oil to make their faces shine, and bread that sustains their hearts.*" Here, we see that food is not only about calories and nutrients but also about joy, strength, and vitality. Each element of God's creation is purposeful, providing the vitamins, minerals, and nutrients we need to live healthy lives.

From a spiritual perspective, the diverse nutrients found in food reflect God's intentional creation, aimed at sustaining life and promoting well-being. The complexity and variety of nutrients found in plants and animals are part of God's divine plan for human flourishing. When we consume food, we are benefiting from the intricate design embedded in creation—a design that supports health, healing, and a life lived in harmony with His purpose. This understanding encourages us to view food as a blessing and to use it in a way that honors our bodies as the temples of God.

Does Food Carry Genetic Information for Wellness?

To understand how food supports our health, it's helpful to understand a bit about DNA. DNA is the genetic code found in all living things—plants, animals, and even us. It's like a set of instructions that tells organisms how to grow and function. When we talk about food carrying genetic information, we mean that the plants and animals we eat have DNA that affects their characteristics—their nutrients, vitamins, and minerals.

When we eat food, we aren't directly consuming DNA in a way that changes our own genetic code, but we are taking in the nutrients that were created according to the DNA of those plants and animals. For example, a fruit or vegetable grows and becomes rich in vitamins because of its genetic makeup. When we eat that fruit, we are benefiting from the nutrients it has produced, which are part of God's design for our health. This is why organic food is unique; it retains all the earth's minerals and vitamins that protect our cells, such as selenium, chromium, and magnesium.

In contrast, genetically modified or processed foods may lack some of these essential earth minerals, compromising their nutritional value and effectiveness in promoting our health. While cooking and digestion break down the physical structure of food, the nutrients remain, and these nutrients are used by our bodies to keep us healthy.

> This is part of God's intricate design—He made plants and animals with all the necessary components to be nourished.

The fact that each type of food has unique nutritional properties that benefit our health points to a Creator who cares deeply about our well-being. However, not all food is equal in terms of nutrition. When we compare natural, organic foods with fast food or heavily processed foods, there are significant differences. Fast food and processed foods often lose many of the natural nutrients that were originally present in the ingredients. The genetic makeup of these foods may still be there, but the way they are processed strips away much of the nutritional value that God intended for us. Additives, preservatives, and artificial ingredients can make fast food convenient, but they do not provide the same quality of nourishment as whole, natural foods.

When we aim to eat healthily, it is important to choose foods that are as close to their natural state as possible — foods that still carry the rich nutrients God designed. By eating organic, whole foods, we align ourselves more closely with the Creator's original plan for nutrition. This not only supports our physical health but also honors the intricate way God made the world to sustain us. Eating foods that retain their natural nutrients helps ensure that we receive the full spectrum of vitamins, minerals, and other compounds that God designed to keep our bodies healthy and strong.

Food and The Body

Food is a gift, a provision, and a tool for connection. It was never meant to be a burden or a source of shame. Throughout Scripture, food is portrayed as a means of fellowship and community. Jesus Himself shared many important moments over meals—whether it was feeding the five thousand with loaves and fishes or breaking bread with His disciples at the Last Supper. Acts 2:46 tells us about the early believers: *"They broke bread in their homes and ate together with glad and sincere hearts."* Food is not just about physical sustenance; it is also about connection. When we share meals with others, we create opportunities for deeper relationships and for showing Christ's love.

> Our bodies are like an earthen suit—a physical garment that God has given us to wear during our time on earth. Just as we take care of our clothes—washing, ironing, and maintaining them to keep them looking presentable—we should also care for our bodies.

Many people spend a lot of money on expensive clothing, meticulously maintaining their appearance, yet often neglect their bodies, which are far more valuable. We treat our physical clothes with care, but sometimes treat our bodies poorly by consuming unhealthy things that damage them. This can make our "suit" wear out sooner, age prematurely, or break down.

We must remember that our bodies are temples of the Holy Spirit and are worthy of care and attention. Proper nourishment is a key part of that care. Food was never intended to harm our bodies but to nourish, sustain, and bring us joy. When we treat our bodies with the same care and respect that we give to our clothes, we honor God's creation and His provision for us. When we treat our bodies as the valuable "earthen suit" that God has entrusted to us, we acknowledge the importance of caring for ourselves physically, spiritually, and emotionally. Our eating habits should reflect this understanding, honoring the body that God has given us while also fostering connection and community with those around us.

Food Significance

Cultural Expression

Food often embodies cultural identity and traditions, acting as a medium through which cultural values, history, and practices are communicated and preserved. In some cultures, sharing food signifies acceptance and safety. Whether it's offering a kola nut, tea, or simply water, each culture has unique customs that convey warmth and belonging. In many of these cultures, when you visit someone's home, they may offer you food, and they anticipate or expect you to receive and eat it. If you don't, it can send a message that you do not accept or trust them.

In many traditional cultures around the world, sharing food is often tied to making agreements or covenants. In some African, Asian, or indigenous cultural practices, accepting food from someone can be seen as forming a pact, and eating carelessly or accepting food in certain contexts can be seen as potentially harmful or spiritually compromising.

However, it is also important to be mindful of the intention behind the food we consume. In many of these cultures, food is not only a symbol of hospitality but can also carry spiritual implications. For instance, in some cultural practices, eating carelessly or without discernment has been associated with spiritual entanglements or even covenants, including demonic covenants. The Bible warns against participating in such practices. In 1 Corinthians 10:20-21, Paul speaks about sacrifices offered to idols being offered to demons, and he urges believers not to partake in these meals, saying, "*No, but the sacrifices of pagans are offered to demons, not to God, and I do not want you to be participants with demons."* Similarly, in 1 Corinthians 11:27-30, Paul emphasizes the importance of discerning the body of Christ when participating in the Lord's Supper, cautioning that failure to do so can lead to judgment. Additionally, Deuteronomy 32:17 highlights the danger of sacrificing to false gods, which reinforces the spiritual risks involved in eating without discernment.

Building Relationships

Sharing food creates a space for connection, conversation, and intimacy. It's a chance to engage with one another on a personal level, reflecting the communal nature of Jesus' teachings. When we sit down to share a meal, we are not just eating to satisfy hunger; we are actively building relationships that foster trust, care, and love. Sharing meals holds profound significance, both socially and spiritually. When we gather around a table, we cultivate deeper relationships and foster community. In the context of Christian faith, this practice can reflect and amplify Christ's love for one another.

Food as Communication

Food can also be a medium of communication that conveys life, death, or spiritual truths. It is not merely sustenance but a means through which we express love, intent (whether good or bad), and commitment. In the Bible, food often carries profound symbolism—like the bread and wine of communion. Similarly, in Ezekiel 3:3 and Revelation 10:9-11, we see examples where men of God are instructed to eat a scroll or book, symbolizing the reception of divine messages that they were then commanded to prophesy.

> It is important to recognize that food has the power to communicate spiritual truths.

This demonstrates how consuming something can carry deep spiritual meaning, shaping one's purpose and message. This means we must be intentional about the meals we partake in, discerning the spiritual implications of the food we consume.

Communion as a Covenant

In the practice of communion, as described in 1 Corinthians 11:23-30, Jesus initiated a sacred act that symbolizes His body and blood. This act transcends mere ritual; it is a profound communication of grace, sacrifice, and unity among believers. Through communion, Christians not only remember Christ's sacrifice but also affirm their relationship with Him and each other.

Communicating Life

When we eat together in a Christ-centered manner, we are not just satisfying hunger; we are communicating life, hope, and love. This reinforces the idea that our meals can be a source of spiritual nourishment and a means to strengthen our faith and relationships. By being intentional in our eating practices, we acknowledge the potential of food to serve as a medium of communication, whether for good or ill. Embracing this understanding can transform our approach to meals, making them a powerful expression of faith and community.

Caution Against Careless Eating

In many cultures, food is tied to rituals and covenants, and engaging in meals without awareness can lead to spiritual entanglements. Some individuals may even experience negative spiritual or physical effects after eating food provided by others, which goes beyond mere food poisoning. This is why it is essential to approach eating with discernment, understanding that the food we consume can have an impact beyond just the physical body.

The Role of Intention

Jesus understood the power of food and its ability to communicate deeper truths. By initiating communion, He highlighted the importance of intention behind our meals. Communion is more than a ritual; it is a profound act that carries the significance of Christ's sacrifice and the unity of believers. In 1 Corinthians 11:30, Paul reminds us of that improper participation in communion can lead to serious consequences: *"That is why many among you are weak and sick, and a number of you have fallen asleep."* This shows us that the act of eating can carry spiritual weight, and being intentional in our eating practices is crucial.

> As we look at food through the lens of God's wisdom, we begin to understand that food is meant to nourish not just our bodies, but also our relationships—with others and with God.

By embracing God's design, practicing moderation, and resisting the temptation to overindulge, we can develop a healthier, more peaceful relationship with food. Remember, God cares about every detail of your life, including what you eat and how you think about food. Let Him guide you as you seek to honor Him in your eating and find true freedom.

3

Rethinking Eating Habits

Rethinking eating habits involves a conscious evaluation and adjustment of how, what, and why we eat. This include mindfulness and intentionality when and how we eat, In Ecclesiastes 10:16-17, these verses provide insight into the importance of wisdom, discipline, and timing, even though it reflection is in leadership, it helped throw in some light to some wisdom and habits around food. This scripture reflects broader themes about how wise choices in daily life—including food and lifestyle—impact overall well-being.

> "Woe to you, O land, when your king is a child, and your princes feast in the morning! Happy are you, O land, when your king is the son of the nobility, and **your princes eat at the proper time, for strength and not for drunkenness!**"

We can apply these principles to our approach towards our food habits, considering the importance of timing, moderation, and intentional lifestyle choices around when, what, and how we eat food. Eating *"at the proper time"* implies making choices that support health and well-being, much like balanced and structured eating patterns that nourish and sustain. These don't necessarily provide an explicit guide to meal structures, however, just mindful and understand the foresight and discipline around food and feasting. Like in the above scripture, the choices of a leader reflect their impact on the community. Wise leaders promote health, including proper eating habits, leading to a stronger, more vibrant society. Similarly, our eating habits can reflect and influence our personal well-being and the people around us.

The Concept of Three Meals a Day

The question often arises: do we really need three meals a day? The practice of eating three meals a day is a long-standing tradition in many cultures, but is it truly necessary for everyone? For some, this pattern works well, while for others, it may not be ideal. The traditional structure of breakfast, lunch, and dinner has been shaped largely by societal norms and historical influences, but modern research suggests that individual nutritional needs can vary significantly. The belief in having three meals a day is more of a cultural norm than a strict nutritional necessity.

Historically, the concept of three meals a day has practical roots. During the 17th century, many people worked in agriculture, which required early rising and long hours of physical labor. To sustain their energy throughout the day, it was crucial to have a substantial meal in the morning—thus, breakfast became an essential start to the day. Later, during the Industrial Revolution in the late 1700s, work schedules became more regimented, with long hours in factories. This led to the reinforcement of three structured meals: breakfast to begin the day, a midday meal to refuel, and dinner to restore energy after work.

> Breakfast was seen as vital to provide energy for the day's labor, while lunch and dinner served to maintain productivity and restore energy.

These eating patterns eventually became cultural norms, especially in Britain, and spread to other parts of the world. The tradition of three meals a day, particularly the emphasis on breakfast, originated from the practical need for energy and sustenance during a time when physical work dictated daily life. Although lifestyles have evolved, this structure remains common in many cultures today, even though it may not be necessary for everyone depending on their individual needs and lifestyle.

Traditional Eating Patterns vs. Modern Needs

Historically, people followed set eating schedules, largely influenced by work routines and family life. The structured three-meal pattern became more prevalent during the Industrial Revolution, as regimented work hours demanded regular mealtimes. Before this, eating habits varied—some cultures ate two larger meals, while others snacked throughout the day. With the shift towards agrarian societies, mealtimes began to align with farming and labor demands, eventually leading to the common practice of three daily meals.

With the changing nature of work and lifestyle today, the rigid three-meal structure may not suit everyone. Some individuals benefit from smaller, more frequent meals to maintain energy and blood sugar levels, while others prefer fewer, substantial meals or intermittent fasting. Imagine if you work from home with less time for any physical activities and you are mostly in front of the computer—why would you eat as much as someone who is working in the field, running up and down, burning a lot of calories? While you may be burning mental energy, the calories burned are not the same. Your eating habits should reflect your energy consumption level, rather than focusing solely on getting full and packing on extra calories. Any unnecessary calories that the body does not use will be stored as fat, leading to weight gain and increasing the risk of obesity.

The key is to listen to your body and choose what is nourishing and life-giving.

Modern dietary trends reflect this flexibility. While some health professionals recommend three meals a day for stability, others advocate for a personalized approach based on individual needs and preferences. Practices like intermittent fasting challenge the traditional meal concept, showing that fewer meals can also support health and well-being. Intermittent fasting involves cycling between periods of eating and fasting, which can help regulate insulin levels, improve metabolic health, and support weight management. Fasting overnight, which naturally happens when we sleep, is also crucial for giving the digestive system time to rest and repair.

> It's particularly important to avoid late-night snacking, as the body doesn't need excess calories while preparing for sleep and rest.

Consuming food late at night, especially high-calorie snacks, can lead to poor digestion, disrupt sleep, and result in unnecessary fat storage, increasing the risk of weight gain and obesity. Ultimately, the idea of three meals a day is more about convenience and tradition than a universal requirement. It's important to understand your own body's needs and choose a pattern that works best for your health and lifestyle.

Recognizing Hunger vs. Boredom

In today's fast-paced world, it's easy to confuse true hunger with boredom or other emotions. Many of us reach for food simply because it's there, because we're feeling restless, or because eating has become a habitual way to pass the time. Learning to distinguish genuine hunger from emotional or boredom-driven eating is crucial for developing a healthier relationship with food.

Identifying Physical vs. Emotional Hunger

True hunger usually builds up over time rather than appearing suddenly. You may experience physical sensations such as a growling stomach, emptiness, light-headedness, or fatigue. When you're genuinely hungry, almost any food sounds appealing—not just particular comfort foods.

> If it's been several hours since your last meal, it's likely that the hunger you feel is real.

Emotional hunger often feels different from true hunger. It may come as a sudden urge without a gradual buildup, typically accompanied by cravings for specific comfort foods that are high in sugar, salt, or fat.

> Emotional eating is often used to fill a void, such as loneliness or restlessness, and can lead to mindless eating—consuming food without paying attention, often while distracted by activities like watching TV.

Strategies to Differentiate and Manage

It's important to recognize patterns in your eating habits. Do you find yourself reaching for food whenever you're bored, stressed, or sad? Identifying these emotional triggers is key to addressing them in healthier ways. One effective strategy is to pause and reflect before reaching for food—ask yourself if you're truly hungry or just bored. Staying hydrated can also help, as thirst is sometimes mistaken for hunger. Engaging in a different activity, like a hobby, a walk, or a quick workout, can help distract you from the urge to eat when you're not actually hungry. Setting regular mealtimes can also help regulate your hunger signals, and practicing mindful eating allows you to fully experience the tastes, textures, and enjoyment of food, which can help prevent overeating. If you are genuinely hungry between meals, opt for healthy snacks that provide real nourishment. By understanding your emotional state, you can make more intentional choices and avoid falling into a cycle of emotional eating.

The Sin of Overindulgence

Honestly, food is something we all love. It brings us joy, it brings us together, and it's something we often turn to for comfort. We celebrate with food—think of birthday cakes, family dinners, and special holiday feasts.

> Food is meant to be a blessing; as Ecclesiastes 3:13 says, *"People should eat and drink, and enjoy the good of all their labor, as a gift from God."*

But sometimes, what's meant to be a blessing can end up being misused, and that can lead to negative effects on our health—physically, emotionally, and spiritually.

Warnings Against Gluttony

Gluttony isn't just about eating too much. It's more than that—it's an attitude of excess and a lack of self-control that ends up shifting our focus away from God. Let's think about it for a moment: have you ever had a bad day and just decided to eat your feelings away? Maybe you grabbed a bag of chips or a tub of ice cream, and before you knew it, you were at the bottom of it. We've all been there. But Proverbs 23:20-21 reminds us, *"Do not join those who drink too much wine or gorge themselves on meat, for drunkards and gluttons become poor..."* It's not that food itself is bad—it's when we use it without any boundaries, when we use it to fill a void that only God can fill, that we run into trouble.

> The problem with gluttony isn't that we love food; it's that we let it take a place in our hearts that belongs to God.

Philippians 3:19 talks about people "*whose god is their stomach*," and it's such a powerful reminder that anything we put above God becomes an idol. When we turn to food for comfort, security, or identity instead of turning to God, it's like we're trying to fill a spiritual hole with something physical. And that doesn't work—it leaves us feeling disconnected, weighed down, and often full of guilt.

> Imagine this: you've had a long, stressful day. You come home and all you want to do is eat something comforting. You open the fridge, grab whatever looks good, and start eating—without really thinking about it. You're not eating because you're truly hungry; you're eating because you want to feel better. And maybe, for a few minutes, it works. But afterward, you still feel empty. Why? Because that emptiness is not the kind that food will fill. But turning to food might seem like a quick fix, but in the end, it's God who offers true comfort and peace.

Gluttony often has deeper roots. It's not just about food—it's about what we're trying to use food to do. Maybe we're feeling lonely, anxious, sad, or overwhelmed. Maybe we've had past experiences that make us fear scarcity, and now we eat whenever we can because we're afraid we won't have enough. Whatever it is, addressing gluttony isn't just about cutting down on food. It's about changing our hearts and allowing God to fill those empty spaces that we're trying to fill with food.

Motives Behind Overeating

There are many reasons—some are physical, others are emotional, and sometimes it's just out of habit. Understanding why we overeat is so important if we want to break free from unhealthy patterns. Sometimes, it's simply because the food tastes amazing, and we want more. Other times, it's because we're trying to comfort ourselves, manage stress, or just distract ourselves when we're bored.

But there can be deeper motives too, like greed or the need to overcompensate. Maybe you find yourself eating without considering those around you, or wanting to eat everything that looks appealing. Sometimes, it's about scarcity—maybe you grew up with limited access to food, and now that you can afford more, you overeat just because you can.

> Emotional triggers like stress, sadness, or loneliness can also drive us to overeat.

When we're feeling drained or depressed, we often turn to food for comfort, hoping it will fill an emotional void that really requires deeper healing. Food can easily become a coping mechanism—it provides temporary relief, but it never truly satisfies our deeper needs. So, it's worth asking yourself: What's your motive? Are you eating because you're truly hungry, or is it because you feel empty, bored, or simply because you can? Recognizing and understanding your motives is a big step toward building a healthier relationship with food.

Food Temptation and Discipline

In Christian teachings, gluttony is one of the seven deadly sins—a vice that leads to overindulgence and a lack of restraint. To overcome gluttony, we need to embrace the virtues that God has given us.

> Galatians 5:22-23 gives us a roadmap: "*But the fruit of the Spirit is love, joy, peace, forbearance (**patience**), kindness, goodness, **faithfulness**, **gentleness**, and **self-control**.*"

These are the tools that show us a sign of what we should bring forth and manifest in our lives.

Self-control is key. It's about learning to pause and ask ourselves why we're eating. Are we genuinely hungry, or are we just giving in to cravings? Self-control, through the help of the Holy Spirit, allows us to make choices that honor God. Proverbs 25:28 says, "*Like a city whose walls are broken through is a person who lacks self-control.*" Without self-control, we leave ourselves vulnerable, but with it, we can create healthy boundaries that lead to freedom.

Gentleness is another important aspect. It encourages us to be compassionate towards ourselves and others. Overcoming gluttony isn't easy, and it's important not to beat ourselves up when we slip up. Instead, we need to recognize that it's a journey, and every step toward greater self-control is progress.

Patience is about resisting immediate gratification. Let's be real—change doesn't happen overnight. Overcoming the habits of overeating takes time. It requires us to trust in God, rely on His strength, and be patient with ourselves along the way.

Faithfulness means staying committed to our well-being, both spiritually and physically. As 2 Peter 1:5-6 says, "*Make every effort to add to your faith goodness; and to goodness, knowledge; and to knowledge, self-control.*" This journey requires effort and commitment, but God is always with us, providing strength through the supply of the Holy Spirit in us.

All of us face food-related temptations. Sometimes it's the urge to eat when we're not really hungry, or to indulge in just a little more even when we're full. But God is faithful. 1 Corinthians 10:13 tells us, *"No temptation has overtaken you except what is common to mankind. And God is faithful; he will not let you be tempted beyond what you can bear. But when you are tempted, he will also provide a way out so that you can endure it."*

> We are never alone in our struggles — God always provides a way out.

Discipline isn't about punishment or deprivation—it's about aligning ourselves with God's will. Hebrews 12:11 tells us, *"No discipline seems pleasant at the time, but painful. Later on, however, it produces a harvest of righteousness and peace for those who have been trained by it."* Discipline is a tool that helps us live in the fullness of God's design, leading to true peace and fulfillment.

This means being mindful of what we eat, recognizing when we're eating because we're truly hungry, and pausing when it's driven by something else. It means inviting God into those moments when we want to turn to food for comfort and allowing Him to be our strength. By leaning on the Holy Spirit and practicing self-control, we can transform our habits and seek fulfillment in God rather than in excess. This is how we honor both our bodies and our spirits, living a life that reflects the true freedom God intends for us.

When to Seek Professional Help

If you're finding it difficult to control unnecessary eating or if food-related habits are impacting your health—physically, emotionally, or spiritually—it may be time to consider seeking support from a healthcare provider or registered dietitian. Professional guidance can offer personalized insights tailored to your unique needs and goals, helping you address the root causes of your eating patterns and make sustainable changes.

Working with a professional, especially one who respects your faith-centered approach, can provide you with tools to become more attuned to your body's signals, such as recognizing true hunger versus emotional cravings. This understanding can empower you to make more mindful choices about when and what to eat, leading to greater well-being and healthier, more balanced habits.

In addition to understanding physical hunger, a trained provider can guide you through managing emotional or stress-related triggers for eating, building strategies to cope without turning to food.

> Seeking help isn't about "fixing" yourself; it's about gaining resources and support to foster a harmonious relationship with food and honoring your body as a gift from God.

Taking this step can lead you toward long-term freedom and peace in your eating journey, allowing you to fully embrace a faith-filled approach to your health.

4

Breaking Free from Food Noise

Effects on Mind, Body, and Spirit

Food noise is that constant chatter in your mind about food—what you should eat, what you shouldn't eat, when you should eat, and the guilt that comes afterward. It can feel overwhelming, and often we don't even realize how much space these thoughts take up in our lives. The truth is, food noise doesn't just impact our physical bodies—it affects our mind, spirit, and even our relationships. Let's break down how.

When it comes to the **mind**, food noise can be exhausting. Think about how many times you've found yourself obsessing over a meal or feeling guilty about what you just ate. These thoughts can drain your energy and distract you from the things that truly matter. It creates a cycle of shame and anxiety, which can negatively affect your mental health over time.

For the **body**, constant overthinking about food can lead to unhealthy patterns. Maybe you overeat to quiet those thoughts or restrict yourself too much in an attempt to feel in control. Either way, your body ends up paying the price.

> Whether it's weight gain, malnutrition, or just feeling tired all the time, the effects of food noise are real, and they can be damaging.

We should also consider the impact food noise has on our relationships with ourselves and others. When we're constantly worried about food, it can lead to feelings of inadequacy and dissatisfaction with ourselves. We might avoid social gatherings or family events because we're too worried about what food will be there. It even affects our finances—overindulging, stress eating, or buying into the latest diet trends or recipes can drain our resources.

Impact on Relationships with God

Spiritually, food noise can affect your relationship with God. If your mind is constantly occupied with thoughts about food, it leaves little room for God's voice. Instead of turning to Him for comfort, we often turn to food, and that keeps us from experiencing the fullness of God's peace. We need to remember that God wants us to be free—not controlled by anything, including food.

Emotional eating is something many of us struggle with, but what if we approached it as a spiritual battle rather than just a physical challenge? When we face those moments of stress, loneliness, or boredom and turn to food, we're often looking for something that food can't truly provide. This is where faith becomes so powerful. We need to recognize that behind emotional eating, there's often a deeper longing—a longing for comfort, peace, or fulfillment. And while food might provide a temporary fix, it's God who offers the lasting comfort we truly need.

Strategies for Managing Food Noise

Breaking free from food noise is possible, but it takes intention and effort. Here are some practical strategies to help manage it and reclaim your peace.

Practical Steps for Control

One of the most effective steps you can take is to acknowledge the noise. It might seem obvious, but many of us don't even realize how much of our mental space food thoughts occupy. Start by paying attention to your thoughts. When you notice food noise, pause and name it for what it is.

> You might think, "*That's just the food noise talking.*" Naming it helps you distance yourself from those thoughts.

Another key step is to invite God into your journey with food. Remember, you don't have to tackle this alone. Pray about your struggles with food and ask God for guidance and peace. When you feel overwhelmed by food thoughts, use it as an opportunity to turn to God. I remember hearing someone on a YouTube video talking about hair care, and she mentioned how she prays about her hair.

> Some people think that's silly, but if God says to ask anything, why not ask about your weight management too? It may sound silly to some, but if it matters to you, then it matters to God. Scripture is full of reminders that God wants us to experience freedom. "*Come to me, all you who are weary and burdened, and I will give you rest.*" (Matthew 11:28, JKV).

It's also helpful to **create healthy routines**. Having consistent meal times and planning balanced meals can reduce the noise by removing uncertainty around food. When you know what and when you're going to eat, you can spend less time worrying and more time living.

> If you're prone to emotional eating, find
> other ways to cope with your emotions.

This could be prayer, journaling, going for a walk, or calling a friend. When we learn to handle our emotions without food, we start breaking the power food noise has over us.

Mindful Eating

Mindful eating is a powerful tool for quieting food noise. It's about being present during your meals—fully experiencing the food you're eating, without distractions or guilt. It may sound simple, but being present while you eat can be transformative. How often do we eat while scrolling on our phones, watching TV, or working on something else? When we're distracted, we don't even taste our food, and we often end up eating more than we need or feeling unsatisfied.

> Eliminating distractions during meals

Start by eliminating distractions during meals. Put your phone away, turn off the TV, and focus on the food in front of you. Notice the colors, smells, and flavors. Take your time, chew slowly, and savor each bite. This practice not only helps you enjoy your food more, but it also allows you to listen to your body's signals—like when you're hungry and when you're full.

Mindful eating is also about avoiding judgment. Many of us label foods as "good" or "bad," and we judge ourselves based on what we eat. But food is just food—it's meant to nourish us, and it's okay to enjoy it. When you're eating, try to let go of the guilt and simply be thankful for the meal in front of you. This doesn't mean we shouldn't care about what we eat, but it does mean that our worth isn't tied to our diet.

> Food is for nourishment, not to be labeled good or bad—enjoy each bite free from guilt and savor gratefully.

Snacking

When can **snacking** be helpful, and when can you consider it better to skip. Snacking can be a healthy way to keep your energy up between meals, especially if you're truly hungry. If you're reaching for a snack just because you're restless, it might be worth finding a different activity to occupy your mind.

> But it's important to pay attention to why you're snacking. Are you eating because your body needs fuel, or are you just bored or stressed?

If you do snack, focus on making it **intentional and healthy**. Try to choose snacks that are nutritious and satisfying, like fresh fruits, vegetables with hummus, or a handful of nuts. These options provide nutrients and keep you feeling full longer. Another great tip is to choose snacks that require **chewing**—things like carrots, apples, or even sugar-free gum. When you're chewing, it sends signals to your brain that you're eating, which can help slow down the urge to keep eating more. It's a simple way to trick your brain into feeling satisfied.

On the other hand, try to **avoid snacking late at night**. Your body doesn't need the extra calories when it's preparing for rest, and late-night snacking can lead to poor digestion and unnecessary weight gain. Instead, if you find yourself wanting something late in the evening, try drinking a glass of water or herbal tea. Sometimes what feels like hunger is actually just thirst or a desire for comfort. Remember, it's about listening to your body and giving it what it truly needs.

By practicing mindful eating, acknowledging food noise, inviting God into your relationship with food, establishing healthy routines, and being intentional about snacking, you can begin to break free from the constant chatter about food.

> The goal isn't perfection; it's progress—learning to listen to your body, nourish it well, and ultimately find your peace in God, not in food.

Trusting God in Overcoming Struggles

One of the first steps in overcoming emotional eating is to acknowledge that it's a struggle and to invite God into that struggle. It's okay to admit that you need help—God wants us to come to Him with our burdens, even the ones that seem small or insignificant.

> When those urges to eat emotionally hit, take a moment to pray.

It doesn't have to be anything fancy; simply say, *"God, I need You right now. I'm feeling overwhelmed, and I don't want to turn to food. Help me find peace in You."* Trusting God means believing that He cares about every part of our lives, including the moments we feel weakest.

When we trust God in our journey, we start to see that we're not alone in our battles. He is with us every step of the way, offering us strength when we feel like we have none left. It's also important to remember that temptation is not a sin—even Jesus was tempted. What matters is how we respond to that temptation. God promises to provide a way out when we're tempted (1 Corinthians 10:13), and sometimes that way out is simply turning to Him in prayer or reaching out to a friend for support. Trusting God in your journey with food means letting go of the idea that you have to do it all on your own. It means being vulnerable enough to ask for His help. I once heard someone say they pray.

5

Fasting, Feasting, and Spiritual Health

Fasting as a Spiritual Discipline

Fasting is a practice that can seem intimidating at first, but it's actually a powerful spiritual discipline that has been part of Christian life for centuries. When we fast, we're not just giving up food—we're making space for God. It's a way to step back from our physical needs and focus on our spiritual needs, drawing closer to Him. Fasting is about surrendering our cravings and saying, "God, You are enough for me." Fasting is truly one of the most powerful tools we have for growing closer to God.

> One of the biggest spiritual benefits of fasting is that it helps us quiet our physical cravings and remind our bodies that we are in charge—not our appetites.

Our bodies often crave things that aren't necessarily good for us, whether it's too much food, unhealthy habits, or other distractions. Fasting allows us to say, "I want what God wants, and I'm going to make sure my body aligns with that." It's a way of training ourselves to put God first, even before our most basic needs.

Think about the story in Matthew 17:14-21, where the disciples couldn't cast out a demon from a young boy. Jesus tells them, *"This kind does not go out except by prayer and fasting."* The point Jesus makes here is powerful—fasting helps us build our spiritual strength and faith. It's not that fasting itself forces God to do something, but rather, it helps us grow in our dependence on Him. It's about being spiritually prepared, about having the faith and courage to face whatever challenges come our way without letting fear or doubt take over.

Fasting also helps us keep our focus on God. When we're fasting, every time we feel that hunger, it's a reminder to turn to God. Instead of letting our cravings control us, we use them as opportunities to pray and lean on God for strength. Imagine how much space that can create in your day—time you can use to pray, read scripture, or simply sit in God's presence without distraction.

> Fasting isn't just about skipping meals—it's about taking the time and energy we'd normally spend on food and investing it in our relationship with God.

Fasting is not about impressing God or earning His favor—He already loves us completely. Instead, it's about removing distractions, realigning our hearts, and focusing on what truly matters. It's about saying, "God, I need You more than anything else." And that's the beauty of fasting—it's a way to put God first, to quiet the noise, and to find our peace in Him.

> Fasting is a way to remind ourselves that we're not just physical beings—we're spir-

itual beings who need God's presence
even more than we need food.

There's no specific formula for fasting—everyone's journey will look a little different. For some, it might mean skipping meals, for others, it might be giving up something like social media or another activity that takes up a lot of their time. The important thing is to use that space to seek God more intentionally and build self-disciple. Whether it's spending extra time in prayer, diving into scripture, or just sitting quietly with God, the goal is to deepen your connection with Him.

Benefits of Fasting

Fasting offers surprising benefits that can profoundly impact both our mindset and overall well-being. Imagine a day without the usual focus on food—no need to plan meals or prepare dishes—and instead, using that time to nurture yourself and deepen your connection with God.

> One of the first things people notice with fasting is the mental clarity and peace that emerge, as it creates space for reflection and spiritual growth.

We'll explore the mental, physical, and health benefits of fasting, focusing on how it can enhance both your mind and body. However, if you have any medical condition that may be affected by fasting, it's essential to consult with your general practitioner before beginning. Ensuring that fasting is safe for you is key to enjoying its benefits fully and aligning with a faith-centered, holistic approach to health.

Mental Benefits of Fasting

One of the mental benefits of fasting is **stress relief**. Many people find that they feel less anxious and more at ease when they're fasting, especially when they use that time to pray or meditate.

> When you fast, your body reduces the production of cortisol, the hormone responsible for stress. It's like your body finally gets a break, and your mind follows suit.

Another benefit is **improved mood**. Some research shows that fasting can actually help lift your spirits, reducing anxiety and depression. It's not a magic pill, but it can help shift your mental state in a positive direction. Of course, everyone is different—some people feel irritable at first when they're hungry, but that often subsides as they continue fasting and start to feel a sense of accomplishment.

> There's something really powerful about telling your body "no" and sticking to it. It gives you a sense of control that spills over into other parts of your life, making you feel stronger and more capable.

Fasting also brings **enhanced mind-body awareness.** When you're not eating, you become more in tune with what your body actually needs, rather than just responding to cravings. You become aware of when you're truly hungry versus when you're just bored or stressed.

> This awareness can be a game changer in understanding your relationship with food and in breaking bad habits.

And let's not forget about **improved thinking**. Many people notice that their thoughts become clearer when they're fasting. By cutting down on excessive carbohydrates and fats, you give your brain a chance to function at its best. You're no longer bogged down by the heavy feeling that comes after eating too much, and you can think with more focus and precision.

Interestingly, fasting also leads to an increase in something called **brain-derived neurotrophic factor (BDNF)**. It's a protein that helps your brain grow new cells and maintain existing ones. There's also something really fascinating about how fasting affects our brain. When you're not eating all day, your brain becomes more alert. You're not constantly bogged down with digesting food, so your mind becomes sharp and clear. As the body produces more BDNF, this means better learning, improved memory, and just feeling more mentally sharp.

> So, when you fast, you're literally boosting your brainpower.

However, it's important to recognize that fasting affects everyone differently. For some, it might bring on negative emotions, like irritability or increased anxiety, especially in the beginning. But for many, these feelings are short-lived, and the long-term benefits far outweigh the initial discomfort. It all comes down to your mindset and how you approach it. If you see fasting as an opportunity to gain control, reduce stress, and draw closer to God, then it becomes much more than just skipping a meal—it becomes a powerful mental and spiritual tool. Fasting isn't just about changing your body; it's about transforming your mind.

> It's about finding peace, clarity, and a renewed sense of purpose. It helps you realize that food isn't your only source of comfort—God is. And when you're able to make that shift, it opens the door to a more meaningful, peaceful, and joyful life.

Physical and Health Benefits of Fasting

Fasting isn't just a health trend—it's something deeply rooted in spiritual practice, and there's a reason why God calls us to fast. **God knows the importance of fasting** for our physical, mental, and spiritual well-being. When we fast, we aren't just nourishing our spiritual lives—we're allowing our bodies and minds to experience a reset that can help us thrive here on earth.

> Fasting can be so powerful for your physical body.

Fasting also helps switch off certain hormones in the body that promote fat storage. When you fast, those fat-making hormones disappear, and your body becomes a fat-burning machine. It's this natural ebb and flow—making fat when we eat and burning fat when we fast—that helps keep us in balance.

One of the physical benefits of fasting is weight loss. When you're fasting, your body starts to burn stored fat for energy. It's simple: when you're not eating, insulin levels drop, and this allows your body to access and burn that fat.

> It's like giving your body permission to finally tap into the energy reserves it's been holding onto.

But fasting isn't just about weight loss—it's also about giving your organs a break. Picture this—our bodies are designed to put on fat when we eat and burn that fat when we're not eating. Think about how much work your pancreas and liver do all day to process all that food. It's like they're constantly working overtime without a break. Fasting allows these organs to rest, reducing stress on your body and helping them function better.

> The problem today? We're rarely giving our bodies that break in between meals because there's always food around us.

We live in a world of abundance, and we're just not getting the downtime our bodies need. For example, many people think a fatty liver is normal because so many people have it, but common doesn't mean normal. Giving your body a break through fasting can help improve liver health and reduce issues like fatty liver. Fasting helps bring back that balance.

Another huge benefit is that fasting encourages autophagy—which is basically a cleaning process your cells go through. It's like taking out the trash in your body. Damaged cells are broken down and recycled, which is super important for overall health. It helps keep your cells young and functioning well, protecting you from age-related diseases like Alzheimer's or even cancer. Speaking of cancer, did you know that cancer cells aren't as efficient as normal cells when it comes to energy production? They rely heavily on glucose. When you fast, glucose levels drop, and cancer cells are the first to struggle—making fasting a powerful tool for reducing the risk of cancer.

Lastly, fasting can also boost your immune system. When you fast, your body produces new white blood cells, strengthening your ability to fight off infections. It's like hitting a reset button on your immune system, making it more effective.

> For those who find fasting tough or feel anxious, there are ways to make it easier. Staying hydrated is key, but don't overdo it—you can have too much of a good thing, even with water.

One trick of staying hydrated is to drink something like bone broth, which has electrolytes that can help you feel like you've had a meal. I've even heard of people using pickle juice or crunching on salt flakes when cravings hit. If you find yourself craving something sweet, sometimes your body actually needs sodium, so this can help!

All these benefits show that fasting isn't just about losing weight—it's about giving your body time to heal, reset, and function the way it was designed to. It's about creating space for both physical and mental clarity, allowing your body to get back into balance, and ultimately live a healthier life. Whether it's weight loss, clearer thinking, or stronger immunity, fasting offers so much for those willing to give it a try.

Detoxification and Types of Fasting

When we talk about detoxification, we're really talking about helping the body do what it's naturally designed to do: cleanse and renew. Fasting can be a powerful way to support this process. By giving the body a break from constant digestion, fasting allows time for rest, healing, and resetting. And the best part? There are different types of fasting to fit various lifestyles, so it's not just about going without food—it's about finding a rhythm that feels balanced and refreshing. Each type of fasting offers its own benefits, helping you feel renewed, both physically and mentally.

Intermittent Fasting

This is a popular one because it's flexible—you decide when to eat and when not to. For example, the 16:8 method means you fast for 16 hours and eat during an 8-hour window. Another option is the 5:2 method, where you eat normally for five days and reduce calories significantly on the other two. The best part? You're not counting calories all the time—you're just being intentional about when you eat.

> During those fasting hours, your body shifts from burning glucose to burning fat, which can help with weight loss and other health benefits. It's like flipping a metabolic switch, allowing your body to work more efficiently.

For those wanting a deeper detox, there's the 24-Hour Fast. This is where you don't eat for an entire day—usually once or twice a week. It sounds tough, but people find it very effective for clearing out their systems. After about 18 to 24 hours, your body enters ketosis, which means it's breaking down fat for energy. It's a great way to give your organs a rest, allowing for deep detoxification and some solid fat burning. It's also a test of mental resilience—by pushing yourself to go without food for 24 hours, you build a stronger sense of self-discipline.

Extended Fasting

This type of fasting usually lasts 48 hours or more. This one's definitely more intense and not for everyone—if you're considering it, it's important to make sure you're doing it safely, ideally with some guidance. Extended fasting takes your body into deeper levels of ketosis and helps with autophagy—the process where your body cleans out damaged cells and regenerates healthier ones. This type of fasting can lead to a profound sense of mental clarity, almost like hitting a reset button on both your mind and body. It's not something you do all the time—maybe once a month or a few times a year—but it can have lasting benefits for your health.

> It is always recommended to seek medical advice especially if you have any underlying medical diagnosis.

When to Fast

The best time to fast depends on your lifestyle and goals. For a lot of people, intermittent fasting is a great way to make fasting a part of their daily routine without it feeling too restrictive. You can choose the time window that fits your schedule. For example, if you're someone who tends to skip breakfast anyway, you might naturally be drawn to the 16:8 method where you start eating at noon. It feels less like a diet and more like a shift in habits.

For those looking for a deeper cleanse or perhaps to kickstart a weight-loss journey, a 24-hour fast once a week could be a good option. It gives your body that needed reset without being too overwhelming. And if you're ready for the next level, extended fasting can help detox your system on a cellular level, which is great for long-term health.

> Fasting isn't just about what's happening in your stomach; it's about what's happening in your entire body and mind.

Detoxification through fasting lets your body rest from the constant digestion it's used to, allowing it to focus on repairing and regenerating. It's like spring cleaning for your insides—getting rid of the old, worn-out cells and making way for new, healthy ones. Whether you're doing a short fast or an extended one, each approach has unique benefits that can help your body, mind, and spirit get back on track.

God's design is perfect, and fasting is one of the gifts He's given us to ensure that our physical, mental, and spiritual selves stay in harmony. He designed us with purpose, and He knows that for us to be successful while we're in these physical bodies, we need balance and discipline.

> It's as if God is saying, "Take a pause. Let go of the distractions. Align your body with your spirit, and let Me speak to your heart."

Through fasting, we become more attuned to God's voice, healthier in our bodies, and clearer in our minds—equipped to fulfill our purpose with strength and focus. It's not just about going without food—it's about making room for what really matters, allowing us to be more effective and live out His will here on earth.

6

Fellowship, Accountability, and Mental Health

Mentorship and Guidance

One aspect that is often overlooked in our journey toward breaking free from food noise is **fellowship and accountability**. We were never meant to walk this journey alone, and that's why mentorship, guidance, and counseling are so crucial. Whether it's about our relationship with food, our mental health, or our faith, we all need someone to help guide us, hold us accountable, and offer professional support when needed.

> In our faith communities, finding a mentor can be a game-changer.

Think about someone who has been where you are and has come out on the other side stronger. Maybe it's an elder in your church, a trusted friend, or someone who has experience dealing with struggles like emotional eating or food addiction. A mentor provides wisdom, support, and encouragement, helping you stay on track and reminding you that your worth is not defined by your struggles with food.

> Finding support in faith communities can take many forms.

Sometimes it's a formal mentorship, other times it's simply being part of a small group that prays for each other, listens, and shares openly. Additionally, seeking counseling from a licensed therapist can provide specialized support for addressing emotional eating, mental health challenges, and the underlying issues that drive unhealthy behaviors. Having people around you who genuinely care and who are also striving to honor God in their lives can make all the difference.

> It's easy to feel isolated when we struggle with food noise or mental health, but the truth is that we're stronger together.

God designed us to live in community because He knows we thrive when we support and uplift each other. It's important to **find a community that empowers you**—people who push you closer to God and encourage you in your journey. Get serious about your God connections, because struggling alone often leads to defeat or being trapped by what we hide. What you expose loses its power over you, and bringing struggles into the light within a supportive community can be incredibly freeing.

Role of Fellowship in Healing

When you're struggling with food noise or emotional eating, it can feel like an overwhelming burden. Sometimes, all you want to do is isolate yourself, but that's where fellowship becomes even more important. Fellowship allows us to break the cycle of isolation and step into the light where real healing can happen.

Accountability is such a powerful tool.

Think of it like this: If you're trying to overcome a bad habit, it's so much easier when you have someone walking alongside you. This is why accountability is such a powerful tool. When you share your goals and struggles with someone, they can help hold you accountable in a loving and supportive way. Whether it's checking in on your progress, praying with you, or even just being there when you need someone to talk to, accountability can help keep you on track.

Breaking free from food noise isn't just about personal discipline—it's about inviting others into the journey. Maybe it's a friend who knows your struggle and checks in on you, or a group from church where you all support each other with your health goals. Knowing someone else is there, cheering you on, and ready to catch you when you fall makes it easier to keep moving forward. James 5:16 says, "Therefore confess your sins to each other and pray for each other so that you may be healed. The prayer of a righteous person is powerful and effective." When we confess our struggles to others and ask for prayer, there's a special kind of healing that takes place.

Diet's Impact on Mental Health

We can't ignore the impact that our diet has on mental health. It's amazing how connected our minds and bodies are. What we put into our bodies doesn't just affect our physical health—it has a huge impact on our emotional and mental well-being too. When we eat foods high in sugar and processed fats, we might feel an initial rush of energy, but it's often followed by a crash that leaves us feeling sluggish, irritable, or even anxious. It's like when you eat a bunch of candy and feel great for about an hour, but then suddenly you're tired, cranky, and maybe even a little sad.

> Our bodies crave balance, and when we feed them the right nutrients, we help support our emotional stability.

On the other hand, foods rich in vitamins, minerals, and healthy fats—like leafy greens, nuts, fish, and berries—can actually help improve mood and mental clarity. Imagine starting your day with a nutritious smoothie packed with fresh fruit, spinach, and healthy fats like avocado. Compare that to starting your day with a sugary donut and coffee loaded with cream and sugar. The difference in how you feel—both physically and emotionally—can be huge. It's not about being perfect, but about making choices that help us feel our best.

> It's also important to remember that food is not the enemy. God gave us food to enjoy, to nourish our bodies, and to bring us together in fellowship.

The problem comes when we use food in ways that it was never meant to be used—like when we use it to numb emotions, distract ourselves, or fill a void that only God can truly fill. When we start seeing food as a tool for nourishment and as a way to honor God with our bodies, it changes our relationship with it.

> If you're struggling with emotional eating, it can help to keep a food journal to track how certain foods make you feel.

Do you notice that you feel more anxious after a day of heavy, processed meals? Or maybe you find that you're more at peace when you've been eating whole, natural foods. Paying attention to the way food affects your mood can help you make better choices for both your body and your mind.

By leaning on mentorship, fellowship, and accountability, and making intentional choices about what we eat, we can begin to break free from food noise and find greater peace in our relationship with food. If there is a need for weight management, it's acceptable to talk to your medical provider to help you jumpstart your journey—whether that means using medication to manage food cravings with the goal of weight loss or working with a nutritionist to plan out your diet and manage your food journey. Additionally, an eating disorder approach that emphasizes understanding the purpose of food and practicing self-love can be incredibly beneficial for recovery and healing.

> We weren't meant to do this alone—God
> placed us in community for a reason.

When we support each other, encourage each other, and lift each other up, we're able to experience healing that goes far beyond what we could do on our own.

7

Conclusion

Transforming Your Relationship with Food Through Faith

As we come to the end of this journey together, remember that finding faith and freedom in your relationship with food isn't about achieving perfection. It's about progress, grace, and allowing God's loving guidance to shape your choices. This journey of transformation is rooted in patience, persistence, and an openness to letting God walk with you every step of the way.

Throughout this book, we've explored how food, faith, and self-care intertwine. Cultivating a healthy relationship with food takes time, but God doesn't expect you to have it all figured out. Instead, He invites you to trust Him as you take small, intentional steps forward. These gradual changes, rooted in faith, can lead to lasting transformation. You now have the tools, insights, and support to make real shifts in your relationship with food.

> When setbacks arise—and they will—remember that resilience, not perfection, is key.

Each day gives you a fresh opportunity to practice mindfulness, offer yourself compassion, and lean into your faith. As you continue on this path, trust that

God is guiding you toward a life where food is no longer a source of control or worry. Instead, it becomes a means of nourishment, joy, and gratitude. You are not alone on this journey; you are part of a larger story of faith, purpose, and renewal. With each small step, you move closer to the life of peace and wholeness that God desires for you.

Steps to Foster a Healthy Relationship with Food as God's Creation

1. **Listen to Your Body:** Start by tuning into your body's natural cues. Notice when you're truly hungry and when you're using food to soothe emotions or fill an emptiness. Pause before you eat, and ask, "Is this hunger, or am I craving comfort?" It's okay to choose differently.

2. **Reframe Your Perspective on Food:** Instead of viewing food as an enemy, see it as a gift from God—a source of nourishment and strength. He created food for us to enjoy, and when we eat mindfully and with gratitude, we honor Him with our bodies.

3. **Seek Fellowship and Accountability:** This journey is not meant to be walked alone. Connect with others—a mentor, a small group, or a trusted friend—who can support your goals and share your struggles. When we open up, we strip power from the things that hold us back, and being part of a community that uplifts and encourages can make a tremendous difference.

4. **Reach Out for Professional Support When Needed:** If you face practical challenges, like weight management or disordered eating patterns, don't hesitate to seek guidance from a healthcare provider or nutritionist. Taking this step is wise and can support your journey. Needing help is not a sign of weakness; it's a commitment to taking care of the body God entrusted to you.

5. **Remember Your True Worth:** Your value does not come from what you eat or how you look—it comes from God. He loves you, values you, and desires peace and freedom for you in all areas of life, including your relationship with food. Some days will feel like victories, and others may feel like setbacks, but know that God's grace is always sufficient. Every small success is worth celebrating, and each challenge is an opportunity to grow.

As you move forward, continue to lean on your faith, God's strength, and the support of those He has placed in your life.

> This journey is about so much more than food—it's about finding freedom, trusting God, and living a life that honors Him in body, mind, and spirit. And that, dear friend, is worth every effort.

And remember: at the end of the book, you'll find three hands-on **Activities with Worksheets** designed to help you deepen your understanding and quiet food noise in practical ways. These include:

- **Quieting Food Noise: Daily Thought Record**
- **Managing Cravings: The 5-Minute Delay Technique**
- **Overcoming Emotional Eating: Emotional Check-In Chart**

These resources are here to guide you through small, purposeful steps toward a peaceful, balanced relationship with food. May each step bring you closer to the joy, peace, and wholeness that God has planned for you. Keep moving forward in faith, and may you experience the fulfillment of living in true freedom.

8

Appendices A - Quieting Food Noise: Daily Thought Record

One of the most effective ways to tackle food noise and emotional eating is by understanding the thoughts that drive our behaviors. The Daily Thought Record is a tool designed to help you identify, challenge, and replace unhelpful thoughts around food. By consistently using this tool, you can develop a healthier mindset and relationship with food, aligned with God's purpose for your body.

How to Use the Daily Thought Record

The Daily Thought Record involves three main steps: capturing your thoughts, evaluating them, and transforming them. This process helps you move from unhealthy thoughts to intentional, nourishing choices. Below, you'll find the template along with examples to guide you through this powerful exercise.

Step 1: Capture Your Thoughts

Each time you find yourself thinking about food—whether it's a craving, a negative thought about your body, or the urge to eat out of boredom—take a moment to write down exactly what you're thinking. Be honest and specific.

> Example: "I need to eat something sweet right now, even though I'm not hungry."

Daily Thought Record Template:

- **Situation**: What happened, or what were you doing when the thought came up?
- **Thought**: What did you think in that moment? Write it down in as much detail as possible.

> Example

- **Situation**: Watching TV after dinner.
- **Thought**: "I deserve a treat. I should get some ice cream."

Step 2: Evaluate Your Thought

Now that you've captured your thought, ask yourself if it's based on truth or if it's driven by an emotional state or habit. Identify if this thought is based on true physical hunger, emotional hunger, or just a habit. Consider if it's helpful or aligns with your health goals and faith-based intentions.

Example: "Am I really hungry, or am I eating because I'm bored? Eating ice cream will make me feel better temporarily, but it's not nourishing my body the way God wants."

Daily Thought Record Template:

- **Emotion**: How did you feel when you had that thought?

- **Reality Check**: Is this thought true or helpful? Does it align with your goal of honoring your body as God's creation?

- **Rating**: Rate how intense this thought or craving is on a scale from 1-10.

Example

- **Emotion**: Bored, restless.

- **Reality Check**: This is not physical hunger. It's an emotional urge.

- **Rating**: 7/10.

Step 3: Transform Your Thought

Replace your unhelpful thought with a positive, intentional thought. Remind yourself of the truth—that God has given you the strength to overcome your cravings and that food is meant to nourish, not to be a coping mechanism.

Example: "I don't need this ice cream to feel better. I can spend time reading, meditating, praying, or doing an activity I enjoy, which will honor my body and my relationship with God."

Daily Thought Record Template:

- **New Thought**: Replace the unhelpful thought with something encouraging and aligned with your health goals.

- **Action Plan**: Write down a positive action you can take instead of eating.

Example

- **New Thought**: "Food is a gift from God meant for nourishment, not to ease my boredom."

- **Action Plan**: Take a walk, read a chapter of a book, call a friend, or spend 10 minutes in prayer.

Daily Thought Record Worksheet

Date	Situation	Thought	Emotion	Reality Check	Rating	New Thought	Action Plan
05/12/24	Watching TV after dinner	"I should get some ice cream"	I feel Bored, restless	This is an emotional urge, not hunger	7/10	"Food is for nourishment, not boredom"	Take a walk, pray, or do some reading

Tips for Success

1. **Keep It Handy**: Print out multiple copies of the Daily Thought Record worksheet or keep a notebook dedicated to these reflections. Keeping it

accessible helps you stay consistent.

2. **Reflect Often**: At the end of each week, look back at your thoughts. See if you notice patterns—are there certain times or emotions that trigger unhealthy eating thoughts? Awareness is the first step to change.

3. **Celebrate Small Wins**: Each time you replace an unhealthy thought with a helpful one, celebrate! You are retraining your mind to think differently, and that's a big deal. Every small step counts.

Quieting Food Noise with God's Help

Remember, this journey isn't one you're taking alone. God is walking alongside you, giving you strength every step of the way. Each time you feel overwhelmed by food noise, lean into prayer and ask for God's wisdom and peace. The Daily Thought Record is just one tool to help quiet that noise, but ultimately, true freedom comes from the One who loves you and wants to see you thrive.

Overcoming Emotional Eating: Emotional Check-In Chart

Emotional eating is a common struggle that many people face. It often happens when we use food to cope with our emotions rather than addressing the root cause of those feelings. The Emotional Check-In Chart is a tool designed to help you understand your emotions, identify triggers, and find healthy, non-food ways to manage what you're feeling. By using this tool regularly, you can develop more mindful eating habits that honor your body and align with God's purpose for your health.

How to Use the Emotional Check-In Chart

The Emotional Check-In Chart guides you through the process of identifying what you're feeling, understanding the root of those emotions, and choosing healthier actions to cope. This simple tool can help you pause, reflect, and make intentional choices about whether you truly need food or if there's another way to care for yourself.

Step 1: Pause and Reflect

Before you reach for food, take a moment to pause and ask yourself, "What am I feeling right now?" Are you actually hungry, or is something else driving your desire to eat? This pause allows you to reflect on your true needs.

Step 2: Identify the Emotion

Use the chart below to identify what emotion you're experiencing. Understanding your emotional state is crucial in making healthier decisions.

Emotion	Feeling Description	Common Triggers
Stress	Overwhelmed, tense, pressured	Workload, deadlines
Sadness	Tearful, heavy, lonely	Loss, rejection
Anxiety	Nervous, worried, uneasy	Uncertainty, fear of failure
Boredom	Restless, unengaged, lacking purpose	Lack of activity, routine tasks
Loneliness	Isolated, disconnected, unloved	Lack of social interaction
Anger	Frustrated, resentful, upset	Conflict, unmet expectations
Happiness	Joyful, excited, content	Success, positive interactions

Step 3: Choose a Healthy Coping Strategy

Once you have identified your emotion, select a non-food action to help you cope with that feeling. The key is to replace the urge to eat with an activity that directly addresses the underlying emotion.

Emotion	Healthy Coping Strategies
Stress	Go for a walk, practice deep breathing, take a hot bath, listen to calming worship music
Sadness	Call a trusted friend, journal about your feelings, pray and meditate on comforting Bible verses
Anxiety	Practice grounding exercises, spend time in nature, focus on slow and controlled breathing, read Scripture
Boredom	Engage in a hobby you enjoy (painting, knitting, playing music), do a small home project, read a book
Loneliness	Attend a church event, join an online faith-based group, connect with a loved one, do something for someone else
Anger	Practice forgiveness exercises, do a physical activity like running or punching a pillow, write a letter (you don't have to send it)
Happiness	Share your joy with someone, engage in a creative activity, offer a prayer of gratitude

Step 4: Write It Down

Documenting your feelings and the actions you take can help you recognize patterns in your emotional eating. Use the following template to log your emotional check-ins:

APPENDICES A - QUIETING FOOD NOISE: DAILY THOUGHT...

Date	Emotion	Trigger	Coping Strategy Chosen	Result
06/15/24	Stress	Work deadline	Went for a 15-minute walk	Went for a 15-minute walk
06/16/24	Boredom	No plans for the evening	Painted for 30 minutes	Felt productive and happy afterwards

Tips for Success

1. Keep It Visible: Print out the Emotional Check-In Chart and place it somewhere you will see it often, like on the fridge or in your journal.

2. Reflect Weekly: At the end of each week, review your entries. Are there emotions that keep coming up? What coping strategies work best for you? Understanding these patterns can help you make long-term changes.

3. Pray and Connect: Invite God into this journey. Prayer is a powerful tool to help us find comfort and peace beyond what food can provide. Ask God to help you see the root causes of your emotional eating and to give you the strength to respond differently.

Finding Comfort Beyond Food

By using the Emotional Check-In Chart, you are making a choice to care for yourself in a more meaningful way. The more you practice this, the easier it will become to reach for God's peace and love instead of a snack.

Managing Cravings: The 5-Minute Delay Technique

Cravings can feel overwhelming at times but managing them is possible with the right tools and mindset. The 5-Minute Delay Technique is a simple but powerful strategy to help you pause, reflect, and ultimately make a more intentional choice about whether or not to indulge in a craving. By using this technique, you give yourself the chance to choose God's purpose for your body over the impulsive desire for immediate gratification. This activity will guide you step-by-step in mastering the technique, so you can effectively handle cravings and build a healthier relationship with food.

How to Use the 5-Minute Delay Technique

The 5-Minute Delay Technique involves delaying action on your craving for just 5 minutes. During this time, you engage in an alternative activity to help you reassess the craving and decide if you truly need or want to indulge. This pause helps break the automatic response to eat and gives you a moment to consider a healthier choice.

Step 1: Recognize the Craving

The first step is to acknowledge that you're experiencing a craving. It might be a sudden urge for a snack, a specific food, or an emotional need disguised as hunger. Once you feel the craving, tell yourself, "I'm craving this, but I'm going to wait 5 minutes before I decide what to do."

> Example: You feel a sudden urge for chocolate after dinner. Instead of grab-

bing it right away, you commit to using the 5-Minute Delay Technique.

Step 2: Set a Timer

Set a timer for 5 minutes. This is your "pause" time where you allow yourself to reflect. During these 5 minutes, don't focus on the food. Instead, engage in a different activity that helps shift your focus.

Suggested Activities During the 5-Minute Delay:

- Drink Water: Sometimes cravings are mistaken for thirst. Drink a glass of water to see if it helps reduce the urge.

- Take Deep Breaths: Practice deep breathing for a few minutes to calm your mind and body.

- Pray or Meditate: Spend a few minutes in prayer, asking for God's guidance to make a choice that honors your body.

- Distract Yourself: Do something you enjoy, such as reading a book, taking a short walk, or listening to uplifting music.

Step 3: Reflect on the Craving

Once the timer goes off, take a moment to reflect. Ask yourself these questions:
- Am I really hungry, or is this just an emotional craving?

- What triggered this craving? Was it boredom, stress, or another emotion?

- How will I feel if I choose to indulge in this craving? Will it bring me closer to my health goals, or will it make me feel regretful?

> Example: You realize that you are not actually hungry; you are just bored and want something to do while watching TV.

Step 4: Make a Choice

After the 5 minutes are up, make a conscious decision. You may decide that you don't need the food after all, or you may choose to have a smaller portion in a mindful way. The goal is not to deprive yourself but to make a thoughtful choice.

> Example: After reflecting, you decide that you don't need the chocolate. Instead, you choose to make a cup of herbal tea, which satisfies you without compromising your goals.

Step 5: Document Your Experience

Writing down your experience can help you track your progress and identify patterns in your cravings. Use the template below to log your 5-Minute Delay experiences:

APPENDICES A - QUIETING FOOD NOISE: DAILY THOUGHT...

Date	Craving	Trigger	Activity During Delay	Final Decision	How I Felt Afterwards
06/20/24	Chocolate	Boredom after dinner	Drank water, prayed	Chose herbal tea instead	Felt proud of making a healthier choice
06/21/24	Chips	Stress after work	Stress after work	Had a small handful mindfully	Felt in control and satisfied

Tips for Success

1. **Start Small:** At first, it may be difficult to delay all cravings. Start by using the 5-Minute Delay for one or two cravings a day. Build up as you become more comfortable with the process.

2. **Celebrate Your Wins:** Every time you successfully use the 5-Minute Delay Technique, celebrate your progress! It takes real strength to pause and make intentional decisions, and every small step brings you closer to a healthier relationship with food.

3. **Keep a Journal:** Use the provided template to track your progress. Over time, you will notice patterns in your cravings, and reflecting on these moments can help you understand yourself better.

Trusting God in the Pause

The 5-Minute Delay Technique isn't just about delaying a craving; it's about creating space for God in that moment. When you pause, you give yourself the opportunity to invite God into your decision-making process. Remember, cravings are often temporary, but the decisions we make can have lasting effects on our health and well-being. With each craving you overcome, you are taking a step toward honoring the body that God has given you. Lean into His strength and trust that He is guiding you towards freedom and health.

9

Appendices B - Daily Thought Record Worksheet

This worksheet is designed as a daily tool to aid you in aligning your thoughts with God's truth. As you use this worksheet, may you not only grow in self-discipline but also find yourself drawing closer to God. It is through aligning our thoughts with His truth that we not only improve our relationships with food but also deepen our spiritual connection with Him.

Daily Thought Record Worksheet

Date	Situation	Thought	Emotion	Reality Check	Rating	New Thought	Action Plan
06/01/24	Watching TV after dinner	"I should get some ice cream."	Bored, restless	This is an emotional urge, not hunger	6/10	"Food is for nourishment, not boredom."	Take a walk, pray, or do some reading.

10

Appendices C- Emotional Check-In Chart

Embarking on this journey is not about achieving perfection; it's about making progress. The Emotional Check-In Chart serves as your guide, helping you to pause, reflect, and choose healthier actions. Each reflection and decision brings you closer to the person God has called you to be—someone who lives in peace, balance, and nourishment of body, mind, and spirit. Let this chart be your companion towards a life where food is seen as nourishment and not an emotional crutch.

The Emotional Check-In Chart

Date	Emotion	Trigger	Coping Strategy Chosen	Result
06/15/24	Stress	Work deadline	Went for a 15-minute walk	Felt calmer and didn't need to snack
06/16/24	Boredom	No plans for the evening	Painted for 30 minutes	Felt productive and happy afterwards

11
Appendices D- The 5-Minute Delay Technique

Use the following template to log your experiences with the 5-Minute Delay Technique. This practice is designed to help you manage cravings more effectively by encouraging you to write down your experiences, track your progress, and identify patterns in your cravings. More importantly, using this technique strengthens your reliance on God for support. Each pause becomes a valuable opportunity to reconnect with your faith, build resilience, and make choices that benefit your mind, body, and spirit.

> As you engage with these worksheets, remember that every step you take is a step toward a more harmonious and fulfilling life. I trust these tools will be invaluable in guiding you along your journey to quiet the food noise.

The 5-Minute Delay Technique

Date	Craving	Trigger	Activity During Delay	Final Decision	How I Felt Afterwards
06/20/24	Chocolate	Boredom after dinner	Drank water, prayed	Chose herbal tea instead	Felt proud of making a healthier choice
06/21/24	Chips	Stress after work	Took a short walk	Had a small handful mindfully	Felt in control and satisfied

Reference

- Anton, S. D., et al. (2018). Flipping the metabolic switch: Understanding and applying the health benefits of fasting. *Obesity*, 26(2), 254-268.

- Fairburn, C. G. (2008). *Cognitive behavior therapy and eating disorders.*

- Foster, R. J. (1998). *Celebration of discipline: The path to spiritual growth.*

- Miller, W. R., & Rollnick, S. (2012). *Motivational interviewing: Helping people change.*

- Olele, I. (2023). Fasting and depression: What to know. *Medical News Today*. Retrieved from https://www.medicalnewstoday.com/articles/fasting-depression

- KJV: Scripture quotations marked KJV are from the King James Version of the Bible (Public Domain).

- Putnam, R. D. (2000). *Bowling alone: The collapse and revival of American community.*

About the Author

NJ Domrufus is more than just an author—she's a compassionate advocate for the human spirit, a mental health professional with a heart for healing, and a dedicated follower of Christ. With a doctorate in psychiatric nursing and extensive counseling experience, NJ has spent her life helping others navigate the complexities of mental health, always leaning into her faith as the cornerstone of resilience and transformation.

In Quiet the Food Noise: Transforming Your Relationship with Food Through Faith, NJ brings her professional expertise and her deeply held beliefs together to offer a powerful and supportive guide for those struggling with their relationship with food. She understands that healing isn't about quick fixes or perfect diets—it's about discovering the grace and freedom that come when we align our lives with God's purpose.

NJ is also a loving wife and mother to two beautiful daughters. She finds joy in the everyday moments of family life, whether it's cooking a favorite meal, travelling, reading or writing a good book, or taking part in community outreach. Her passion for service extends to her work as the founder of the Gifted Orphan Foundation (GOF), where she dedicates her time to providing care and support for orphaned children.

NJ believes in the importance of nurturing the soul and finding moments of grace in the everyday. Her writing is both practical and deeply personal, filled with the wisdom that comes from walking beside others in their times of need. Her love for writing comes from a desire to connect, to uplift, and to build others up.

ABOUT THE AUTHOR

NJ's books are an invitation—an invitation to find hope, to seek support, and to embrace the journey of healing, no matter how challenging it may seem. Through her words, she offers readers the chance to quiet the noise, reconnect with God, and rediscover the joy that lies in nourishing both body and soul.

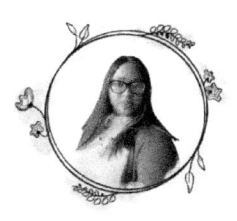

More Books by The Author

- Navigating Grief with God: *Finding Hope After Loss*

- Guarding Your Soul Gates: *Protecting Your Heart and Mind as a Believer*

- Decline the Offer: *Rejecting Negative Whispers with God's Truth*

- The Discovery Journey (Children's book story for ages 7 to 10 years of age)

- The Beatitudes Book Series (Children's 9 books story series for ages 4 to 9 years of age)

- Adventure Book Series (Children's 9 books story series for ages 4 to 10 years of age)

- How Doctors Take Care of You: A Visit to Dr. Kind's Clinic (Children's book story for ages 4 to 9 years of age)

- Brave Like David: *Facing Giants with Kindness* (Coloring Book)

- Anchored in His Love Journal: *A Journey of Grace and Wisdom*

MORE BOOKS BY THE AUTHOR

- Anchored in His Love Journal: *A Journey of Grace and Wisdom* Anchored in His Love: *Daily Meditation for Women* (a Meditation book for Women, designed to help you connect with God in a meaningful way, even on the busiest of days, featuring scripture, reflections, and inspiration to deepen faith.)

- Strength for Today: *30 Days of Faith and Peace for Anxious and Heavy Hearts*

Look for these titles in stores and online soon!

Printed in Great Britain
by Amazon